Keto Meal Prep

Easy Ketogenic Diet Recipes for Beginners

Jerryk luna

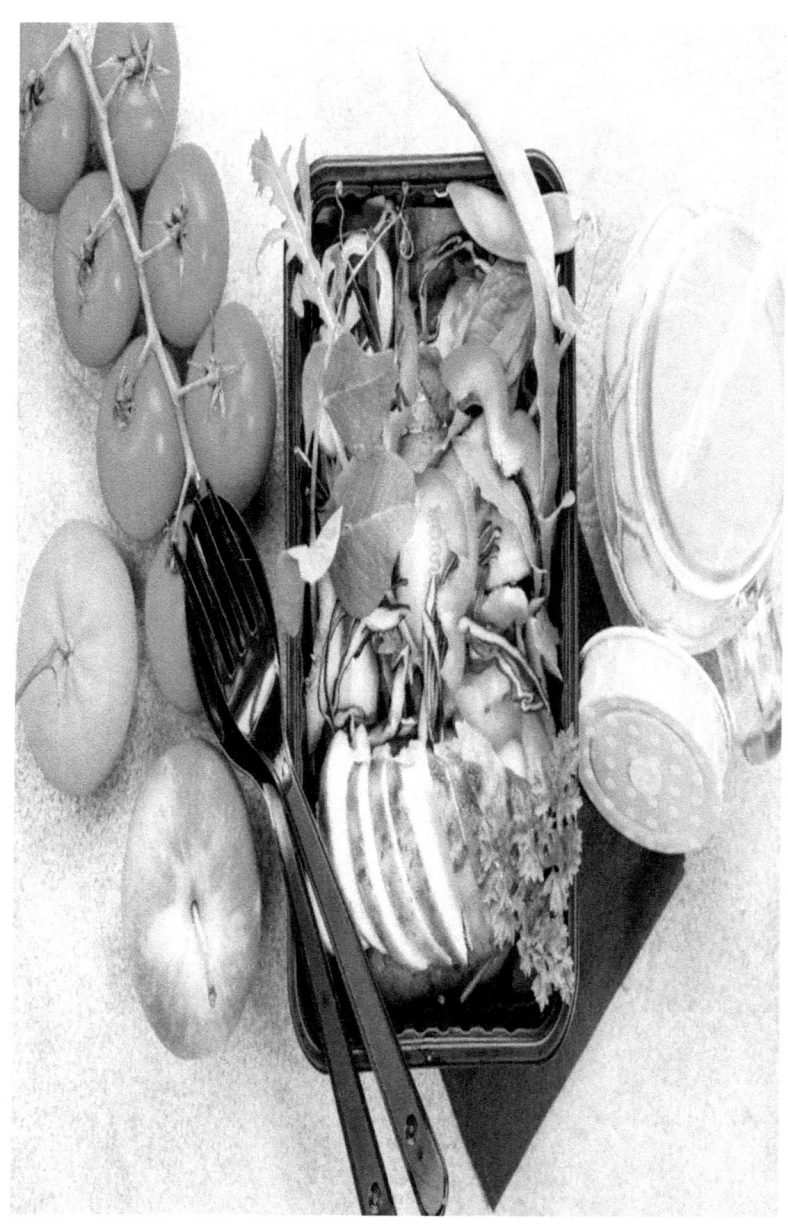

or backing by the trademark owner. All trademarks and brands within this book are for clarifying purposes only and are the owned by the owners themselves, not affiliated with this document.

Table of Contents

Introduction

I want to thank you and congratulate you for downloading the book, "Keto Meal Prep: Easy Ketogenic Diet Recipes for Beginners" Top 60 Delicious and quick & easy keto recipes for you.

In this book you will learn about the benefits of the keto diet, the keto diet pantry essentials, necessary kitchen equipment, you will find a keto-friendly food list and tips to improve the success of the keto diet. Not just this, but there are 60 easy to cook and testy recipes given in this book that will help you prepare delicious keto-friendly meals within no time.

Ketogenic Diet for Beginner

What is Ketogenic Diet?

The Ketogenic diet, also referred to as the keto diet or low carb high fat (LCHF) diet, refers to a type of low carbohydrate diet that is high in fat and adequate in protein.

The diet has one priority; to get the body into optimal ketosis i.e. a state where the body relies on ketones for energy as opposed to glucose. For this to happen, you have to ensure that your intake of carbohydrates is very low (not more that 50grams) then pair the low carbohydrates intake with high fat intake and moderate protein intake.

This way of eating, as you might have noticed, goes against everything you've ever been taught about eating healthy i.e. you should eat more of carbohydrates, take minimal amount of fats and a moderate amount of proteins- according to the USDA food pyramid. And it is for a reason; the huge amount of carbohydrates that you've been taking over the years are primarily the reason why you are unhealthy and overweight/obese.

Benefits of the keto Diet

The keto diet is one of the most popular diets these days and rightly so. The ketogenic diet is a high fat and a low crab diet. The idea of this diet is to shift your body into a state of ketosis and hence the name of this diet.

The primary source of fuel for the human body is glucose. The body produces glucose and the primary source of energy fats. During ketosis, the body starts to burn fats instead of glucose to provide power. In this section, you will learn about the different benefits of the ketogenic diet.

Basic Keto Guidelines

The keto diet works by, in a way, flipping around the food pyramid that we are used to seeing in classrooms and doctor's offices. While our standard food pyramid has grains as one of the most consumed items and oils and fast at the very tip, the ketogenic diet almost entirely eradicated grains and carbohydrates, while natural fats make up a large portion of the diet's base.

In the ideal percentage breakdown for the keto diet, 75% of your energy should be coming from natural fats, 15-25% should be coming from protein, and <5% should be coming from carbohydrates. 0% should come from sugar. The lesser carbohydrates, the better. For a lot of people, this can be rough at first. After all, glucose and carbs have become our most defaulted to sources of energy. It takes out bodies time to make the switch to relying on ketones instead. But as it is with intermittent fasting, the longer you go without sugar and carbs, the less your body will actively crave them.

Keto practitioners usually see a very basic assortment of food in their diet.

These include natural fast and oil, eggs, meat, fish, vegetables that grow above ground and some fruit.

Foods to generally be avoided during keto are most fruits, candy of any kind, beer, juice and soda, refined carbohydrates, root vegetables and rice.

Keto is so different from how most of us are used to eating because the starchy foods that have become our default dietary staples of the years are not allowed. This is similar to the Paleo diet, with the main differences being the energy percentage breakdown, and that may processed foods are keto-friendly. But otherwise, the tow diets are very much alike.

Quick Tips you can follow

- Keto is a simple, straightforward diet routine but you need to know the basics before you jump into it.
- How do you cook easy keto meals?
- I have been avoiding fats all these years, how do I get it back to my diet?
- My work routine often forces me to eat out once in a week. How do I manage to stay on keto then?
- How do I start my day on a keto diet?

These common questions might pop up when you are following the diet for the first time. It is quite simple to get started with keto – no complication at all!

- You can consume eggs in any form; however, it is best to add more coconut oil, olive oil and butter while preparing the eggs.

- You do not necessarily need to start your day with a mandatory breakfast. No, it is not really the important meal of the day- breaking the fast, (breakfast) is important. So, if you are not hungry in the morning, you do not need to eat for the sake of eating. Drink lots of water, have a cup of herbal tea or a cup of coffee. You often experience reduced hunger when you are on keto, so skipping a meal is fine!
- If you are someone who wakes up with a grumbling stomach every morning, not to worry there are tons of easy-to-make breakfast recipes available. You can get hold of a few in this book too!
- Plan your main meals (Lunch and Dinner) much ahead of time. A simple main course made of meat or fish accompanied by a vegetable side or a salad. Or a super nutritious vegetable main with a healthy smoothie should do the magic!
- If you feel constantly hungry when you start the keto diet, eat more fat and fiber-rich food – eggs, leafy green, cruciferous veggies, etc.
- If you are out at an official dinner party or a get-together with your friends, replace your pasta or bread with veggie mains + olive oil or butter.
- Go for a fish-based dish or replace the high-carb food with extra mixed vegetables. Try the egg-based meals scrambled eggs, omelet, fried eggs, etc.
- Choose the burgers without buns and replace your French fries with veggies and add a bit of cheese or guacamole to it.
- Mexican dishes offer extra salsa, cheese and cream.
- Choose berries with cream, mixed cheese board as your dessert option.

Breakfast

Slow Cooker Breakfast Meatloaf

Serves: 4 pic per person

Ingredients

- ½ teaspoon sea salt
- ½ teaspoon paprika
- ½ teaspoon black pepper
- 1 teaspoon dried thyme
- 1 teaspoon ground sage
- 1 teaspoon red pepper flakes
- 1 teaspoon dried oregano
- 1 teaspoon fennel seeds, ground
- ½ garlic powder
- 4 tablespoons almond flour
- 1 egg
- 1lb. ground pork
- 1 cup diced onion
- ½ tablespoons coconut oil

Directions

1. At medium-low heat, soften that onion in a tablespoon of oil until transparent. Then remove from heat and let cool.
2. Add all the ingredients to a large bowl apart from the ground pork. Stir or whisk to blend.
3. Add in the softened onions and the ground pork to the bowl and combine the ingredients manually using your hands.
4. Then pick the meat mixture and put in the center of the crockpot's insert. Shape it into a loaf and position it half an inch from the side of the insert.

5. Once done, put the top the loaf and close the crockpot's lid. Cook the meatloaf on low for 3 hours, or until the internal temperature is 150 degrees F.
6. Then let the meatloaf cool for up to 30 minutes after turning off the crockpot and removing the lid to make it easier to remove the meatloaf. Move to a separate dish.
7. You can serve immediately or keep it refrigerated overnight and serve for breakfast. To serve, simply reheat the slice at medium low heat for minute or two.

Nutritional Information Per Serving: Calories 410, Fat 28g, Carbs 5g, Protein 32g

Cheese and Mushroom Strata

Serves 3 per person

Ingredients

- 1/8 teaspoon salt
- ½ tablespoon Dijon
- 1 tablespoon thyme, finely chopped
- 11/4 cups milk
- 4 eggs
- 1 cup grated gruyere cheese
- Keto friendly bread, cut into 1-inch pieces
- 21/2 thick slices
- 1/2 – 227g package cremini mushrooms sliced
- ½ tablespoon Olive oil

Directions

1. Over medium-high heat, melt oil in a non-stick frying pan. Add in mushrooms and cook for about 5-6 minutes, or until the mushroom are tender and their liquid evaporated.
2. Using a large piece of coil, line the bottoms and sides of a Crockpot. Lightly coat with oil.
3. Cover the bottom with a third of the bread then scatter the mushrooms over the bread.
4. Sprinkle the mixture with a third of the cheese, and then add half of the remining bread, and the rest of mushrooms and cheese. Add the remaining bread on top.
5. At this point, beat eggs with Dijon, thyme and milk in a large bowl. Pour the mixture over the bread and season with fresh pepper.
6. Carefully press down the bread to soak into the mixture and topwith cheese. Cook on low for 8 hours.

7. Once set, open the lid and allow to stand for 15 minutes. Remove the foil that holds the strata using oven mitts
8. Move the dish to a serving dish and serve with a favorite salad.

Nutritional Information Per Serving: Calories 191, Carbs 20g, Protein 14g, Fat 5g

Keto Zucchini Breakfast

Servings: 2 per person

Ingredients

- 1 zucchini diced
- ½ avocado
- ½ cup mushrooms chopped
- 1 tablespoon chives parsley chopped
- 1 garlic clove
- ¼ teaspoon salt
- 1 tablespoon coconut oil

Directions

1. Add the chopped onion to the hot oil and sauté until translucent and completely off-liquid.
2. Add the minced garlic and mix well until the raw flavor goes off.
3. Add the chopped mushrooms are tender and cooked thoroughly.
4. Continue to stir the contents until they turn slightly brown
5. Now, add the diced zucchini to the pan and continue to cook for another 15 minutes until the entire contents are thoroughly cooked.
6. Seven with salt and mix once more. Remove from heat and top it with parsley and avocado.
7. Transfer to a plate and serve warm.

Nutritional Information Per Serving: Calories 150, Carbs 10g, Protein 17g, Fat 6g

Matcha Keto Smoothie Bowl

Servings: 1 per person

Ingredients

- 1 teaspoon matcha powder
- 1 tablespoon coconut flakes
- 1 tablespoon chia seeds
- 8 ounces coconut yogurt
- 1 tablespoon cacao nibs
- 1 tablespoon goji berries

Directions

1. Blend together the coconut yogurt and matcha powder on high for 60 seconds until creamy and smooth.
2. Transfer the smoothie into a bowl
3. Top it with coconut flakes, chia seeds, cacao nibs and goji berries
4. Serve immediately.

Nutritional Information Per Serving: Calories 110, Carbs 5g, Protein 12g, Fat 4g

Cheesy Thyme Waffles

Servings: 4 per person

Ingredients

- ½ large head riced cauliflower
- 2 green onion stalks
- 1 c. of each:
- Packed collard greens
- Finely shredded mozzarella cheese
- 2 large eggs
- 1/3 c. parmesan cheese
- 2 t. freshly chopped thyme
- 1 tbsp. of each:
- Olive oil
- Sesame seeds
- ½ t. for each
- Salt
- Ground black pepper
- 1t. garlic powder

Directions

1. Prepare the cauliflower in a food processor until it reaches a crumbly texture.
2. Toss in the thyme, spring onion, and collard greens, pulsing to combine well.
3. Transfer the mixture to a mixing container, add the remaining fixings, then mix well again. Spoon it over the waffle iron and cook until done.
4. Arrange on a serving dish and enjoy with your favorite toppings.

Nutritional Information Per Serving: Calories:201g, Carbohydrates:5g, Protein 13g, Fat 15g

Deviled Eggs for Brunch

Servings: 3 per person

Ingredients

- 6 large boiled eggs
- ¼ cup yellow mustard
- 1 tbs. mayonnaise
- 1 cup paprika
- Garnish: parsley/salt/pepper

Directions

1. Boil the eggs and cool
2. Mix the egg yolks with the rest of the ingredients.
3. Stuff the eggs. Sprinkle with your chosen condiments as desired.

Nutritional Information Per Serving: Calories:266g, Carbohydrates:2g, Protein 18g, Fat 21g

Fried Queso Fresco

Servings: 2 per person

Ingredients

- 1 tablespoon coconut oil
- 1-pound queso fresco
- ½ tablespoon olive oil

Directions

1. Chop the cheese into either rectangles or cubes.
2. Heat both of the oils to the smoking point and then add the cheese.
3. Fry the cheese on each side and then flip until it's thoroughly brown.
4. Remove and let the cheese rest to cool and drain using the towels to remove the oil.

Nutritional Information per Serving: Calories: 280g, Carbohydrates: 6g, Protein:8g, Fat:21g

Blueberry Yogurt Smoothie

Servings: 2 per person

Ingredients

- Blueberries-10
- Yogurt- 0.5 Cup
- Vanilla extract- 0.5 teaspoon
- Coconut milk – 1 cup
- Stevia – As need

Directions

1. Add all of the fixings into blender, mixing well.
2. When creamy, pour into 2 chilled mugs.

Nutritional Information per Serving: Calories: 265, Carbohydrates: 3g, Protein:4g, Fat:6g

Black Greek Eggs

Servings: 1 per person

Ingredients

- Sun dried tomatoes – 0.25 cup
- Feta cheese – 0.5 cup
- Oregano – 0.5 teaspoon
- Chopped kale – 1 cup
- Eggs – 12

Directions

1. Warm up the oven to reach 350-degree F.
2. Cover a baking tin with foil and a spritz for nonstick cooking spray.
3. Whisk the eggs and combine with the rest of the fixings. Stir into the prepared pan. Bake for 25 minutes.
4. Transfer to the countertop to completely cool slice.
5. Store in the refrigerator for 4-5 days in an airtight container.
6. You can also place them into individual portions.

Nutritional Information per Serving: Calories: 105, Carbohydrates: 5g, Protein:8g, Fat:4g

Zoodle Chicken Soup

Servings: 2 per person

Ingredients

- Chicken broth – 3 cups
- Chicken breast – 1
- Avocado oil – 2 tablespoons
- Green onion – 1
- Celery stalk – 1
- Cilantro – 0.25 cup
- Salt for taste
- Peeled zucchini – 1

Directions

1. Chop or dice the breast of the chicken. Pour the oil into a saucepan and cook the chicken until done. Pour in the broth and simmer. Chop the celery and green onions and toss inti the pan. Simmer for 3-4 more minutes.
2. Chop the cilantro and prepare the zucchini noodles. Use a spiralizer or potato peeler to make the noodles Add to the pot.
3. Simmer for a few more minutes and season to your liking.
4. Store in a glass container in the fridge it will remain testy for 2-3 days.

Nutritional Information per Serving: Calories: 305, Carbohydrates: 6g, Protein:35g, Fat:17g

Pizza Waffles

Servings: 2 per person

Ingredients

- 4 large eggs
- 6 tablespoons almond flour
- 2 tablespoons bacon grease
- 1 cup keto friendly tomato sauce
- 28 slices pepperoni
- ½ cup Parmesan cheese, grated
- 2 tablespoons psyllium husk powder
- 2 tablespoons baking powder
- Salt for taste
- Pepper powder for taste
- 6 ounces cheddar cheese, shredded

Directions

1. Add eggs, almond flour, bacon grease, Italian seasoning, tomato sauce, Parmesan cheese, Psyllium husk powder, baking powder, salt and pepper into a blender and blend until smooth.
2. Preheat the waffle iron. Pour ¼ of the mixture. Cook until done.
3. Repeat with the remaining batter to make 3 more waffles.
4. Spread ¼ cup tomato sauce on each waffle. Sprinkle cheese. Place pepperoni slices if using.
5. Place waffles in a preheated oven and broil until cheese melts.

Nutritional Information per Serving: Calories: 601, Carbohydrates: 15g, Protein: 32g, Fat: 50g

Vegan Keto Porridge

Servings: 2 per person

Ingredients

- ¼ cup coconut flour
- 4 tablespoons keto friendly vegan vanilla powder, unsweetened
- Erythritol to taste
- 6 tablespoons golden flaxseed meal
- 3 cups almond milk, unsweetened

Directions

1. Add coconut flour, protein powder and flax meal into a saucepan and stir.
2. Pour almond milk and stir. Place over medium heat. Stir constantly until thick.
3. Add sweetener and stir.
4. Add sweetener and stir.
5. Ladle into bowls and serve with keto friendly toppings of your choice.

Nutritional Information per Serving: Calories: 247g, Carbohydrates: 18g, Protein: 16g, Fat: 12g

Blackberry chocolate shake

Servings: 2 per person

Ingredients

- 2 cups coconut milk, unsweetened
- 4 tablespoons cocoa powder
- ½ teaspoon xanthan gum
- Ice cup blackberries
- 20-25 drops liquid stevia
- 4 tablespoons MCT oil

Directions

1. Gather all the ingredients and add into a blender.
2. Blend for 30-40 second or until creamy. Add water to dilute the smoothie if desired.
3. Pour into a glass and serve with crushed ice.

Nutritional Information per Serving: Calories: 342, Carbohydrates: 14g, Protein: 4g, Fat: 6g

Green Smoothie

Servings: 2 per person

Ingredients

- 4 cup spinach or kale leaves
- 4 Brazil nuts
- 2 scoops Greens powder
- 2 tablespoons psyllium husk powder
- 20 almonds, chopped
- 2 cups chilled coconut milk from carton
- 2 scoops whey protein powder

Directions

1. Gather all the ingredients and add into a blender.
2. Blend for 30-40 second or until creamy. Add water to dilute the smoothie if desired.
3. Pour into glasses and serve.

Nutritional Information per Serving: Calories: 375, Carbohydrates: 15g, Protein: 14g, Fat: 28g

Low Carb Chocolate Almond Smoothie

Servings: 1 per person

Ingredients

- 1 cup almond milk
- 1 tablespoon cacao powder
- ¼ cup ice
- 2 tablespoon almond butter
- 1 half of avocado
- Stevia, to taste

Directions

1. Place the avocado in the high-speed blender.
2. Pour the almond milk and add the ice to it.
3. You can add stevia if you want it sweet else you can skip the step.
4. Blend the contents on high for 60 second until smooth
5. Add the almond butter and cacao powder to the mixture.
6. Blend again on high for 45 seconds until creamy and smooth
7. Transfer to a glass and serve chilled.

Nutritional Information per Serving: Calories: 310, Carbohydrates: 12g, Protein: 10g, Fat: 18g

Chocolate Strawberry Smoothie Bowl

Servings: 1 per person

Ingredients

1. 4 tablespoons cacao powder or cocoa powder.
2. ¼ cup chopped walnuts
3. 1.5 cups almond milk
4. 4 scoops collagen protein
5. 3 cups ice
6. Stevia drops to taste
7. 2 large strawberries
8. Stevia sweetened chocolate shavings to garnish
9. Strawberry slices to garnish

Directions

1. Add all the ingredients except collagen into a blender.
2. Blend on high for 50-60 seconds or until smooth.
3. Add collagen and pulse for 2-3 second until just combined.
4. Pour into bowls. Serve with chocolate shavings and strawberry slices.

Crispy Pork Bites

Servings: 1 per person

Ingredients

- 21 ounces thin pork belly strips
- 1 medium onion, chopped
- ½ cup heavy whipping cream
- Pepper powder to taste
- 3.8 ounces blue cheese, crumbled
- 2 teaspoons fine salt for taste.

Directions

1. Place pork strips in a baking dish. Sprinkle salt over it and rub it into it. The pork strips should have a thin layer of salt over it.
2. Bake in a preheated oven at 450-degree F for about 30-45 minutes or until golden brown in color and crisp. Be careful after 30 minutes as it can burn. Remove from the oven.
3. Meanwhile, place a pan over medium low heat. Add butter. When butter melts, add onions and cook until golden brown.
4. Increase the heat to medium and stir in cream. When cream is warm enough, add blue cheese and mix well.
5. When cheese melts, increase heat to high heat. Let it heat for a couple of minutes. Turn off the heat and transfer into a serving dish.
6. Serve crisp pork with cheese dip.

Nutritional Information per Serving: Calories: 440 g, Carbohydrates: 2 g, Protein: 19 g, Fat: 40 g

Tomato Asiago Soup

Servings: 8 per person

Ingredients

- 2 cans tomato paste
- 1.5 cups Asiago cheese, shredded
- 2 teaspoons dried oregano
- Salt for taste
- Pepper powder to teste
- 2 cup water
- 2 teaspoons garlic, minced

Directions

1. Place a soup pot over medium heat. Add tomato paste, garlic and onion. Mix well.
2. Add cream and whisk well.
3. When it begins to boil, add cheese, a little at a time and whisk well each time.
4. Add water and let it boil for about 5 minutes.
5. Ladle into soup bowls. Sprinkle pepper on top and serve.

Nutritional Information per Serving: Calories: 300 g, Carbohydrates: 10 g, Protein: 8 g, Fat: 12 g

Ginger Snap Cookies

Servings: 1 per person

Ingredients

- ¼ cup unsalted butter
- 1 large egg
- 2 cup almond flour
- ½ teaspoon ground cinnamon
- 1 tablespoon vanilla extract
- ¼ teaspoon ground cloves
- ¼ teaspoon nutmeg
- ¼ teaspoon Salt

Directions

1. Set the oven temperature to 350-degree F.
2. Whisk the dry components in a mixing bowl. Blend in the rest of the ingredients into the dry mixture using a hand blender.
3. Measure the dough for approximately 9 to 11 min. or until it's brown.

Nutritional Information per Serving: Calories: 74 g, Carbohydrates: 2 g, Protein: 2 g, Fat: 6 g

Slow Cooker Bread Pudding

Servings: 4 per person

Ingredients

- 1 tablespoons raisin
- ½ teaspoon cinnamon
- 1.5 teaspoon vanilla extract
- ¼ cup swerve
- 1 egg white
- Whole egg
- 1.5 cups almond milk
- 4 slices pumpkin bread

Directions

1. Cut the keto bread into pieces. Then mix all the ingredients in the crockpot.
2. Cook the mixture on high heat until the liquid is soaked up by the bread, or for 4 to 5 hours.

Nutritional Information per Serving: Calories: 180 g, Carbohydrates: 12 g, Protein: 7 g, Fat: 3 g

Lunch or Dinner

Keto Swedish Meatballs

Servings: 4 per person

Ingredients

- 1 tablespoon Dijon mustard
- 1 tablespoon Worcestershire sauce
- 1.5 cups heavy (whipping) cream
- 1.5 cups chicken broth
- 4 tablespoons salted butter
- ¼ teaspoon allspice
- 0.5 teaspoon ground nutmeg
- ¼ cup diced onions
- 1 tablespoon water
- 1 Egg
- 1 cup mild cheddar cheese, shredded
- 1lbs. ground meatloaf blend

Directions

1. Preheat your oven to 400 degrees F. Meanwhile, set a slow cooker to the low setting.
2. Using parchment paper, line a large baking pan and set aside.
3. Mix together allspice, nutmeg, water, onion, egg cheddar cheese and ground meat.
4. Roll the mixture in 1-and-a-half inch meatballs and layer them onto the baking pan.
5. Bake the meatballs for around 20 minutes. Alternatively, wait until the thermometer reads 140 degrees F.
6. As the meat cooks, heat butter in a small skillet over medium heat along with chicken broth and heavy cream.

7. As soon as it starts to simmer, lower the heat to low and simmer for another 20 minutes while stirring frequently.
8. Once the sauce reduces in half, add in Worcestershire sauce and the mustard. Then transfer the sauce in a slow cooker along with the meatballs.
9. Cook the mixture for 2 hours on low for the meatballs to marinate.
10. Stir after 30 minutes and serve not beyond 2 hours of cooking.

Nutritional Information Per Serving: Calories 770, Carbs 5g, Protein 70g, Fat 45g

Keto Slow-Cooker Beef & Broccoli
Servings: 4 per person

Ingredients

- 1 red bell pepper
- 1 head broccoli
- ½ teaspoon salt
- ¼ -1/2 teaspoon red pepper flakes
- 3 garlic cloves, minced
- 1 teaspoon freshly grated ginger
- 3 tablespoon your sweetener
- 1 cup beef broth
- 2/3 cup liquid aminos
- 2-pound flank steak
- 1 teaspoon sesame seeds, optional

Directions

1. Begin by setting the slow cooker to the low setting. Then proceed to slice a flank into chunks.
2. Once hot, add the steak, salt, pepper, garlic, sweetener, beef broth and coconut amines to the crockpot.
3. Cook the ingredients for about 4 to 6 hours. Meanwhile, prepare bell pepper and broccoli. Simply slice the bell prepper into 1-inch pieces and chop the broccoli to florets.
4. Once cooked, stir the steak then add in red pepper and chopped broccoli. Cook for about 1 hour until crisp, and then toss the mixture together.
5. At this point, sprinkle with sesame and serve garnished with sesame seed if you like it. You can also serve over cauliflower rice.

6. If need be, thicken the sauce using arrowroot thickener. Just combine 2 tablespoons of water with a tablespoon of arrowroot thickener and add to the steak mixture once cooked through. Add enough of it until you achieve desired consistency.

Nutritional Information Per Serving: Calories 420, Carbs 14g, Protein 64g, Fat 15g

Veggie Frittata

Servings: 2 per person

Ingredients

- 2 cup baby spinach
- 1 chopped avocado
- 1 chopped tomato
- 1 minced garlic clove
- ¼ diced onion
- 6 eggs
- ½ tablespoon nutritional yeast
- 3 tablespoons avocado oil
- ½ teaspoon ground cumin
- 2 tablespoons coconut milk
- ¼ teaspoon chili powder
- Sea salt and black pepper for test.

Directions

1. Preheat oven to 350 degrees Fahrenheit.
2. Grease a small baking dish with a bit of coconut oil and set aside
3. Crack the egg into a medium-sized bowl and add the salt, pepper, chili powder, coconut milk, ground cumin and nutritional yeast.
4. Whisk together the contents in the bowl until the mixture turns frothy
5. Heat the remaining coconut oil over medium-high heat in a skillet.
6. Add the onions and garlic to the hot oil.
7. Season with pepper and salt. Stir-fry until the contents turn fragrant as you continue to mix well.

8. Add the avocado to the onion-garlic mixture and sauté for 5 minutes.
9. Now add the baby spinach and stir well until the spinach wilts
10. Transfer the sautéed vegetables to the greased baking dish and top it with the chopped tomato.
11. Pour the egg mixture over the tomato and mixed veggies until the contents are covered with the mixture
12. Bake for 25 minutes until the contents are cooked well and the eggs puff up.
13. Remove from the oven and wait for it cool.
14. Transfer the veggie frittata to a plate and serve warm.

Slow Cooked Beef & Red Wine Stew

Servings: 4 per person

Ingredients

- ½ fresh flat-leaf parsley, chopped
- ½ tablespoon butter, unsalted
- ½ cup dry red wine
- 2 tablespoons tomato paste
- Fresh Black pepper
- Kosher salt
- 11/2-pound pot roast, trimmed and cut into 4 pieces
- ½ tablespoon canola oil
- 3 sprigs thyme
- 2 cloves garlic, chopped
- 1 large celery rib, chopped
- ½ chopped large red onion
- ½ package of cremini mushrooms
- ½ pound carrots or rutabaga cut into small pieces
- ½ teaspoon Dijon mustard
- 1.5 tablespoon coconut or almond flour
- 1 cup beef stock

Directions

1. In a crockpot, whisk together mustard, flour and beef stock. Add in thyme, garlic, celery, onion mushrooms and carrots.
2. In a large skillet, heat oil over medium heat then season the beef with pepper and salt.
3. Cook for 10-12 minutes or until browned, while turning occasionally.

4. Transfer the ingredients to a Crockpot. To the skillet, add in tomato paste and cook for a minute, stirring.
5. Add wine add cook for 30 seconds while scrapping up the browned bits. Transfer to a Crockpot.
6. Discard the thyme. Take out the beef and use two forks to shred it. Return to crockpot and stir in butter.
7. Cover and cook for 5-6 hours on high or 7 to 8 hours on low. Once tender, serve while topped with parsley.

Nutritional Information Per Serving: Calories 450, Carbs 20g, Protein 45g, Fat 30g

Grilled Chicken Skewers with Garlic Sauce

Servings: 4 per person

Ingredients

For the Skewers

- 1 Pound chicken breast, cut into large cubes (approximately 1-inch)
- 1 Onion, chopped
- 2 bell peppers, chopped
- 1 Zucchini

For the Garlic Sauce

- 1 head garlic, peeled
- 1 teaspoon salt
- approximately¼ cup lemon juice
- approximately 1 cup olive oil

Additional ingredients for the marinade

- ½ cup olive oil
- 1 teaspoon salt

Directions

1. Heat up the grill to high.
2. Place the garlic cloves and salt into the blender. Then add in around 1/8 cup of the lemon juice and ½ cup of olive oil.
3. Blend well for 5-10 seconds, then slow your blender down and drizzle in more lemon juice and olive oil alternatively until you hear the blender sound shift a

bit. The consistency will then change into mayo-like consistency. If it doesn't work, don't worry – the sauce won't look amazing, but it'll still taste good!

4. Keep 1ST half the garlic sauce serves with. Take another half of the garlic sauce and add in the additional ½ cup olive oil and teaspoon of salt. Mix well – this makes the marinade.

5. Chop the chicken, onion, bell peppers, and zucchini into approximately 1-inch cubes or squares. Mix them in a bowl with the marinade.

6. Place the cubes on skewers (usually, we grill on the bottom for a few minutes to get the charred look and then move the skewers top top rack with the lid down to cook the chicken well)

7. Serve with the garlic sauce you kept.

Nutritional Information Per Serving: Calories:570, Carbohydrates: 15g, Protein 40g, Fat 30g

Greek Chicken &Vegetable Ragout

Servings: 2 per person

Ingredients

- Fresh Pepper
- 1/3 cup chopped fresh dill
- 1/3 cup lemon juice
- 2 large egg yolks
- 1 large egg
- ½ ounce can artichoke hearts, rinsed
- ¾ teaspoon salt
- 4 cloves garlic, minced
- 1/3 cup dry white wine
- ½ ounce can chicken broth, reduced-sodium
- 2 pounds boneless, skinless chicken thighs, trimmed
- 1-pound rutabagas, 1-inch-wide wedges
- 3 cup baby carrots

Directions

1. Spread the rutabagas and the carrots over the slow cooker. Then arrange the chicken over them.
2. Over medium-high heat, bring salt, garlic, wine and broth to simmer in a medium saucepan.
3. Pour the broth mixture over the vegetables and chicken and cover the cooker. Cook for about 4 to 4.5 hours on low or 2.5 to 3 hours on high.
4. As soon as the veggies are tender and the chicken is cooked through, add artichokes, cover and cook for 5 minutes on high heat.
5. Meanwhile, in a medium bowl, whisk lemon juice, egg yolks and egg until well incorporated.

6. Using a slotted spoon, move the veggies and chicken to a serving boil. Cover to remain warm.
7. At this point, ladle ½ cup of the cooling liquid into lemon mixture and whisk until smooth. Whisk the mixture into the liquid that remained in the Crockpot.
8. Cover and cook for about 15-20 minutes while whisking occasionally. Remove from heat after the sauce is slightly thickened and has reached a temperature of 160 degrees F.
9. Stir in pepper and dill, and now pour the sauce over the veggies and chicken.

Nutritional Information Per Serving: Calories 320g, Carbs 25 g, Protein 31 g, Fat 9 g

Creamy Tomato Basil Chicken Pasta

Servings: 2 per person

Ingredients

- 2 chicken breasts, cubed
- 2 Tablespoon ghee or coconut oil to cook in
- 1 can diced tomatoes (400g)
- ½ cup basil, chopped
- ¼ cup coconut milk
- 6 cloves garlic, minced
- Salt to taste
- 1 zucchini, shredded for the pasta

Directions

1. Sauté the chopped chicken in the ghee or coconut oil until cooked.
2. Add in the can of chopped tomatoes and add in salt. Place on a simmer and cook the liquid down.
3. In the meantime, prepare the pasta. If using zucchinis, shred them in the julienne peeler or a spiralizer. If using spaghetti squash, slice it in half, remove the seeds, cover lightly with some coconut oil and microwave each half for 7 minutes.
4. Add the basil, garlic and coconut milk to the chicken and cook for 5 minutes longer.
5. Place half of the pasta into each bowl and top with the creamy tomato basil chicken.

Nutritional Information Per Serving: Calories:440 g, Carbohydrates:20 g, Protein:58 g, Fat 22 g

Pan-Fried Pork Tenderloin

Servings: 2 per person

Ingredients

- 1-pound pork tenderloin
- Salt and pepper to taste
- 1 Tablespoon coconut oil

Directions

1. Cut the 1-pound pork tenderloin in half
2. Place the 1 tablespoon of coconut oil into a fry pan on a medium heat.
3. After the coconut oil softens, place the 2 pork tenderloin bits into the pan.
4. Once that side is cooked, turn using tongs to cook the other sides. Keep cooking until the pork looks cooked on all sides.
5. Cook all sides of the pork until the meat thermometer shows an internal temperature of just below 145F or 63C
6. The pork will keep on cooking a bit afterward you take it out of the pan.
7. Let the pork site for a few minutes and then into 1-inch thick slices with sharp knife.

Nutritional Information Per Serving: Calories:344, Carbohydrates:10g, Protein 40g, Fat 25g,

Beef Curry

Servings: 2 per person

Ingredients

- 1-pound beef round or other boneless cut, cut into 1-inch cubes.
- 1 medium onion, sliced
- 1 Tablespoon curry powder
- 1 Teaspoon ground cumin
- 1Teaspoon ground coriander
- 1Teaspoon ground turmeric
- 1 Teaspoon cardamom
- ¾ cup of coconut milk
- 2 carrots sliced
- 1 bell pepper, diced
- 10 button mushrooms
- 1 Tablespoon fish sauce
- 1 teaspoon freshly grated ginger
- 2 cloves garlic, minced
- ¼ cup fresh basil leaves, chopped
- Salt to taste
- Coconut oil to cook in

Directions

1. In a pan, sauté the beef and onions in coconut oil on medium heat for 4-5 minutes until the beef is browned.
2. Add the spices, coconut milk, carrots, bell peppers, mushrooms, and fish sauce. Take to the boil, then cover and simmer for 50 minutes until the beef is tender.
3. Add the chopped basil, garlic, ginger, and salt to taste and simmer for 10 more minutes.

Nutritional Information Per Serving: Calories:440, Carbohydrates:11g, Protein 25g, Fat 33g, Sugar: 2g Fiber: 4g

Creamy Keto Fish casserole

Servings: 4 per person

Ingredients

- 25 ounces of white fish
- 15 ounces broccoli
- 3 ounces butter + extra
- 6 scallions
- 11/4 cups heavy whipping cream
- 2 tablespoon small capers
- 1 tablespoon dried parsley
- 1 tablespoon Dijon mustard
- ¼ teaspoon black pepper
- 1 teaspoon salt
- 2 tablespoons olive oil
- 5 ounces leafy greens chopped, for garnishing

Directions

1. Preheat the oven to 400 degrees Fahrenheit
2. Heat the oil in a pot over medium-high heat.
3. Fry the broccoli florets in the hot oil for 5 minutes until tender and golden.
4. Transfer the fried florets to a small bowl and season it with salt and pepper. Toss the contents to ensure all the florets get the equal amount of seasoning.
5. Add the chopped scallions and capers to the same saucepan and fry for 2 minutes. Return the florets to the pan and mix well.
6. Grease a baking tray with a little amount of butter and spread the fried veggies in the baking tray.
7. Add the sliced fish to the tray and nestle it among the veggies.
8. Mix the heavy cream, mustard and parsley in a small bowl and pour this mixture over the fish-veggie mixture.

9. Top this with the remaining butter and spread gently over the contents using a spatula.
10. Bake for 20 minutes until the fish is cooked thoroughly and the cream and butter melt lusciously.
11. Transfer to a plate and garnish with chopped greens. Serve warm and enjoy!

Spinach and Mozzarella Frittata

Servings: 3 per person

Ingredients

- ½ onion
- 1 cup 2% shredded mozzarella cheese
- 1 cup olive oil
- 6 egg
- 2 cup milk
- ½ white pepper and black pepper
- Salt to test
- 1 diced tomato
- 1 cup packed baby spinach

Directions

1. Chop and removed the stems from the spinach and dice the onion.
2. Add the oil to a small skillet using the med. Heat setting and saute the onion for about 5 minutes.
3. Spray the cooker with the oil spray.
4. Combine ¾ of the cheese and the rest of the cheese and the rest of the ingredients in a mixing container and add the slow cooker. Sprinkle the residual cheese on top of the egg combination.
5. Secure the lid and cook under the low setting for 1-1 ½ hour. Eggs should be set.

Nutritional Information Per Serving: Calories: 141g, Carbohydrates: 4g, Protein 12g, Fat 8g

Keto Chicken wings with creamy broccoli

Servings: 4 per person

Ingredients

For the baked chicken wings

- 3 pounds chicken wings
- ¼ teaspoon cayenne pepper
- ½ orange, zest and juice
- 2 teaspoons ground ginger
- ¼ cup olive oil+ extra
- 1 teaspoon salt

For the creamy broccoli

- 25 pounds broccoli chopped
- ¼ cup fresh dill chopped
- 1 cup mayonnaise
- Salt and pepper for taste

Directions

1. Preheat the oven to 400 degrees Fahrenheit.
2. Take a small bowl and place the orange zest in it. Add the cayenne pepper, ground ginger and salt to the zest. Pour the orange juice and the oil to the contents, Mix thoroughly and set aside.
3. Place the chicken wings in a plastic zip bag and pour the prepared orange zest marinade into the plastic bag.
4. Shake the bag until the marinade mixes well with the chicken. Refrigerate the marinated chicken for 15 to 20 minutes.
5. Grease a baking tray with extra olive oil and place the marinated chicken wings in single layer.
6. Bake for 45 minutes in the middle rack of the oven until the chicken is thoroughly cooked and browned.

7. Meanwhile, boil the broccoli florets in salted water for 10 minutes until they soften a bit.
8. Strain the boiled broccoli and transfer it to a blow. Add the mayonnaise, dill, salt and pepper to the bowl. Mix well and set aside.
9. Transfer the cooked chicken to a serving plate and add the creamy broccoli over it. Serve warm and enjoy!

Lobster Salad

Servings: 4 per person

Ingredients

- ¼ cup melted butter
- 1-pound cooked lobster meat
- ¼ cup mayonnaise
- 1/8 cup black pepper

Directions

1. Chop the lobster into bite-sized pieces.
2. Melt and empty the butter over the lobster.
3. Gently toss the lobster and then blend in the mayonnaise with the pepper.
4. Chill in a covered dish for a minimum of 10 minutes.

Nutritional Information per Serving: Calories: 300g, Carbohydrates: 1.5g, Protein: 21g, Fat:23.4g

Keto Salad

Servings: 4 per person

Ingredients

- 2 eggs
- ½ red onion chopped
- 3 ounces turnip
- 2 ounces cherry tomatoes
- 7 ounces green beans
- 7-ounce romaine lettuce
- 2 ounces olives
- 2 garlic cloves
- 2 tablespoons olive oil
- Salt and pepper, to taste
- 2 tablespoons small capers
- ½ cup olive oil
- ½ tablespoon Dijon mustard
- 1 minced garlic clove
- 1 tablespoon fresh parsley
- ¼ cup mayonnaise
- Juice of ½ lemon

Directions

1. Place the capers in a high-speed blender and add the Dijon mustard mayonnaise, parsley and garlic clove to it.
2. Blend on high for 60 seconds until smooth.
3. Pour the olive oil and lemon juice to the blended mixture and blend again for 30 seconds until creamy and smooth
4. Transfer the dressing to a bowl and set aside.
5. Boil the eggs, peel the shell and cut them into wedges. You can soft boil the eggs.
6. Cut the peeled turnips into half-inch pieces and parboil them in lightly salted water for 5 minutes in a small pan

7. Parboil the trimmed green beans in lightly salted water for 5 minutes in another pan.
8. Rinse the boiled beans and turnip in cold water and set aside.
9. Heat the oil in a frying pan over medium-high heat and fry the green beans in it.
10. Add garlic, pepper and salt to the beans in the pan. Stir-fry until cooked through
11. Place the lettuce leaves on a plate and add the tomatoes, onion, egg wedges, fried beans, boiled turnip and olives.
12. Drizzle the dressing over it and serve immediately.

Falafel with Tahini Sauce

Servings: 2 per person

Ingredients

- 1 cup raw pureed cauliflower
- ½ tablespoon ground coriander
- 1 tablespoon ground cumin
- ½ cup ground slivered almonds
- 1 teaspoon kosher salt
- 1 minced garlic clove
- ½ teaspoon cayenne pepper
- 2 large eggs
- 2 tablespoon freshly chopped parsley
- 3 tablespoons coconut flour

Ingredients for the Tahini Sauce

- 4 tablespoon water
- 2 tablespoon tahini paste
- 1 teaspoon salt
- 1 minced garlic clove
- 1 tablespoon lemon juice
- Olive oil

Directions

1. Puree enough cauliflower to make one cup with a grainy texture. Process the almonds the same way, but don't over-grind. Combine the ingredients in a mixing bowl and add the remaining fixings until it's well blended.
2. Warm up about half of the olive oil. Make 3 patties and add to the pan.
3. Cook until it's brown and then flip 4 minutes for each side should be sufficient. Add them to a platter for the oil to drain.

4. Mix all of the tahini components in a bowl and then add a little water at a time until it reaches the desired consistency.
5. Serve with the tahini sauce with a garnish of tomato and parsley.

Nutritional Information per Serving: Calories: 280g, Carbohydrates: 6g, Protein:9g, Fat:23g

Rainbow Salad

Servings: 8 per person

Ingredients

- White balsamic vinegar – 0.5 cup
- Olive oil – 2 tablespoons
- Minced garlic cloves – 2
- Chopped parsley – 0.25 cup
- Salt & Pepper – 1 pinch
- Chopped red cabbage – 2 cups
- Assorted salad greens – 8 cups
- Chopped cucumber – 1 cup
- Raw sunflower seeds – 0.5 cup
- Diced red bell pepper – 1

Directions

1. Whisk all of the dressing fixings together. Pour into a serving container.
2. Drain the chickpeas and prep the veggies. Prepare the salad.
3. Put the salad in individual dishes and pour on the dressing. If you used a jar, just shake.

Nutritional Information per Serving: Calories: 111g, Carbohydrates: 14g, Protein:16g, Fat:8g

Cinnamon Apples

Servings: 4 per person

Ingredients

- Brown sugar – 0.5 cup
- Sugar – 0.5 cup
- Cinnamon – 1 tablespoon
- Nutmeg – 0.125 teaspoon
- Unsalted butter – 2 tablespoons
- Cornstarch – 3 tablespoons
- Granny smith apples – 6
- Salt – 1 pinch

Directions

1. Peel and slice the apples thin.
2. Combine all of the fixings in the instant pot. Press the manual function for 18 minutes. Natural release the pressure 10 minutes and open the pot.
3. Stir and serve or prep.
4. Note: The macro totals are calculated using regular sugar and brown sugar.
5. Let the apples cool to room temperature. Store in an airtight container or heavy-duty freezer bags.
6. Refrigerate for up to 7 days.
7. You can keep the apples fresh in the freezer for about 2 months.

Nutritional Information per Serving: Calories: 108g, Carbohydrates: 3g, Protein: 11g, Fat: 2g

Lemonade Fat Bombs

Servings: 2 per person

Ingredients

- Cream cheese – 4 oz.
- Butter – 2 oz.
- Lemon zest & juice – 0.5 of 1 lemon.
- Swerve – 2 tsp
- Pink Himalayan salt – 1 pinch or to taste.

Directions

1. Take the butter and cream cheese out of the fridge and let it become room temperature before using. Zest the lemon and juice it into a small dish.
2. In another container, mix the butter with the cream cheese. Use a hand mixer to combine all of the fixings until well mixed.
3. Spoon the mixture into small molds or cupcake paper liners in a muffin tin pan.
4. Stick the chosen holder in the freezer for two hours.
5. Take them out of the molds and put them in a zipper-top baggie to enjoy any time.
6. Store in the freezer for up to three months.

Nutritional Information per Serving: Calories: 402g, Carbohydrates: 6g, Protein:6g, Fat:41g

Testy Short Ribs

Servings: 4 per person

Ingredients

- Keto-friendly soy sauce – 0.25 cup
- Beef short ribs– 6 to 4 oz.
- Rice vinegar – 2 tablespoons
- Fish sauce – 2 tablespoons
- Red pepper flakes – 0.5 teaspoon
- Sesame seeds – 0.5 teaspoon
- Onion powder – 0.5 teaspoon
- Minced garlic – 0.5 teaspoon
- Ground ginger – 1 teaspoon
- Salt – 1 tablespoon.
- Cardamom – 0.25 teaspoon

Directions

1. Mix the fish sauce, vinegar, and alternative soy sauce.
2. Arrange the ribs in a dish with high sides. Add the sauce and marinate for up to 1 hour.
3. Combine all of the spices together. Take the ribs from the dish and sprinkle with the rub.
4. Warm up the grill and cook for 3 to 5 minutes on each side.
5. Put the ribs in a platter to cool.
6. Put the ribs in a platter to cool.
7. Place in freezer bags or into plastic containers until it's time to serve.

Nutritional Information per Serving: Calories: 680g, Carbohydrates: 5g, Protein:24g, Fat:60g

Chicken Kinu

Servings: 2 per person

Ingredients

- Breasts of chicken – 2
- Cloves of garlic – 2
- Butter – 4 tablespoons
- Green onion – 1 stalk
- Parsley – pinch
- Tarragon – pinch
- Pepper and salt – to taste
- Pork rinds – 1 oz.
- Coconut flour - 0.25 cup
- Egg – 1

Directions

1. Set the oven temperature to 350-degree F.
2. Use a tenderizing hammer to pound the chicken until they are approximately one-half-inch to one-inch thick. Flavor it with the tarragon, pepper, salt, and parsley.
3. Add chopped bits of butter, garlic, and green onion evenly to the pieces of chicken. Close with toothpicks.
4. Crush the pork rinds for the crumbs.
5. Make dredging dishes, one each for flour, a beaten egg, and the pork rind crumbs.
6. Cover the chicken with the flour, egg, then the rinds. Close them tightly with a toothpick. Let the fixings chill in the fridge for about ½ hour.
7. Fry the breasts until browned on all sides in a lightly oiled pan.
8. Transfer and arrange them in a baking dish.
9. Bake for approximately 20 minutes. Baste with any leftover butter.

10. Let the chicken cool completely. Store in the fridge for one days.
11. You can also portion the fixing into freezer bags and store for later.
12. When ready to serve, add to a bed of lettuce.

Nutritional Information per Serving: Calories: 515g, Carbohydrates: 505g, Protein:55g, Fat:30g

Chicken and Blueberry Salad

Servings: 2 per person

Ingredients

- 20 blueberries
- 2 large bag salad leaves
- 4 teaspoons lemon juice
- 4 tablespoons coconut oil
- 1 small onion, sliced
- 4 tablespoons olive oil
- 2 large chicken breasts, chopped
- Salt for taste
- Pepper for taste.

Directions

1. Place a skillet over medium heat. Add coconut oil. When it melts, add chicken and cook until tender. Sprinkle salt and pepper and stir.
2. Transfer into a serving bowl. Add blueberries, salad leaves, onion, olive oil and lemon juice.
3. Divide into 2 bowls and serve.

Nutritional Information per Serving: Calories: 490, Carbohydrates: 5g, Protein: 27g, Fat: 42g

Pan Fried Cod

Servings: 4 per person

Ingredients

- Ghee – 3 tablespoons
- Cod fillets – 4
- Minced garlic cloves – 6
- Garlic powder – shake
- Salt – 1 pinch

Directions

1. Melt the ghee and add help of the garlic into a skillet.
2. Arrange the fillets in the pan using med-high heat. Sprinkle with the garlic pepper and the salt.
3. Once it turns white halfway up its side, turn it over and add the remainder of the minced garlic.
4. Continue cooking until it flakes easily.
5. Store a day or warp up in foil and add to a plastic freezer bag for a longer time.
6. When ready to eat, serve with some ghee/garlic from the pan.

Nutritional Information per Serving: Calories: 162, Carbohydrates: 6g, Protein: 8g, Fat: 5g

Servings: 4 per person

Ingredients

For salad:

- 6 tablespoons olive oil
- Fresh grounded pepper for taste
- 2 tablespoons lemon juice
- 2 head romaine lettuce, chopped
- ½ red onion, finely sliced
- 1 cucumber, sliced
- ½ cup fresh parsley, chopped

For Chicken:

- 4 chicken breasts, chopped into cubes
- 2 teaspoons paprika
- 2 tablespoons garlic powder
- ¼ teaspoon cayenne pepper
- 8 tablespoons avocado oil
- 2 teaspoons cumin powder
- 2 tablespoons onion powder
- 2 teaspoons Italian seasoning
- Salt to teste

Directions

1. To make dressing, add all the ingredients of dressing into a bowl and whisk well.
2. To make chicken, add paprika, garlic powder, cayenne pepper, cumin, onion powder, Italian seasoning and salt into a bowl and stir.
3. Add chicken and toss until chicken is well coated with the spice mixture.
4. Place a skillet over medium heat. Add oil. When the oil heats, add chicken and cook until done.

5. Remove chicken with a slotted spoon and place on a plate lined with paper towels.
6. To make salad, add all the ingredients of salad into a serving bowl. Drizzle dressing over it. Toss well.
7. Top with chicken and serve.

Nutritional Information per Serving: Calories: 740g, Carbohydrates: 15g, Protein: 55g, Fat: 45g

Keto Buns
Servings: 6 per person

Ingredients

- 2 cups almond flour
- 6 tablespoons psyllium husk powder
- 3 teaspoons baking powder
- 2 teaspoons sea salt
- 3 teaspoons cider vinegar
- 11/2 cups boiling water
- 4 egg whites Garnish
- 3 tablespoons sesame seeds
- 2 tablespoons butter

Directions

1. Preheat the oven to 300-degree F
2. Combine the dry fixings in a large mixing bowl.
3. Add the boiling water, egg whites and vinegar to the bowl and beat the ingredients with a hand mixer for 30 seconds. Ensure that the consistency of the dough resembles Play-Doh.
4. Line a baking tray with parchment paper.
5. Moisten your hands and divide the dough into six pieces.
6. Place the six pieces on the prepared baking tray, and place the tray in the lower rack in the oven.
7. Bake for 60 minutes. When the timer goes off, tap the bun at the bottom. If you here a hollow sound, they are done.
8. Serve warm with butter.

Sausage and Cabbage Melt

Servings: 4 per person

Ingredients

- 4 spicy Italian chicken sausages
- 2 tablespoon coconut oil
- ½ cup diced onion
- 1.5 cup purple
- 1.5 cup green
- 2 tablespoon chopped fresh cilantro
- 2 slices Colby jack cheese

Directions

1. Remove the sausage casings and rough-chop them. Shred the cabbage and chop the onions.
2. Add the coconut oil, cabbage, and onion in a large skillet using the medium-high setting for approximately 8 minutes. The veggies should be tender.
3. Blend the cheese and cover. Turn the heat off and let it rest for 5 minutes for the cheese to melt.
4. When it is time to serve, stir gently and add the cilantro.

Nutritional Information per Serving: Calories: 235g, Carbohydrates: 8g, Protein: 19g, Fat: 12g

Keto Nutty Fat Bombs

Servings: 6 per person

Ingredients

- ½ tablespoon black sesame seeds
- ½ teaspoon turmeric powder
- 3 scoops MCT oil powder
- A pinch Chinese 5 spice powder
- 5 drops liquid stevia
- ¼ teaspoon cinnamon powder
- A pinch pepper powders
- 3 tablespoons warm water

Directions

1. Add oil powder, spices and sesame seeds into a bowl and stir.
2. Stir in the warm water. Mix until well incorporated.
3. Divide the mixture into 6 small silicone molds.
4. Place molds in the freezer until it sets.
5. Remove from the molds and serve it.

Nutritional Information per Serving: Calories: 80 g, Carbohydrates: 3 g, Protein: 2 g, Fat: 6 g

Keto Caprese omelet

Servings: 6 per person

Ingredients

- 6 eggs
- 5 ounces mozzarella cheese
- 3 ounces cherry tomatoes cut in halves
- 2 tablespoon olive oil
- 1 tablespoon basil
- Salt and pepper for taste

Directions

1. Take a mixing bowl and crack the eggs into it. Add salt and pepper to the cracked eggs.
2. Whisk together using a form until well combined.
3. Add the basil to the whisked egg and mix well.
4. Slice the cheese and keep aside.
5. Heat the olive oil in a large pot over medium heat.
6. Add the cherry tomatoes to the hot oil and fry for 3 minutes until cooked through
7. Pour the egg mixture over the tomatoes and let it cook for a while.
8. When the egg is slightly firm, add the cheese slices over the top.
9. Reduce the heat and let the omelet cook until it is completely set.
10. Transfer to a plate and serve hot.

Pork and cabbage Casserole

Servings: 6 per person

Ingredients

- 1 small green cabbage
- ½ ounce pork rinds, crushed
- ½ pound ground pork
- ½ small onion, finely chopped
- 1 small egg
- ½ stalk celery, finely chopped
- ¼ teaspoon ground nutmeg
- 3 cubes chicken bouillon, made into broth
- 1.5 tablespoons soy sauce
- 1 bay leaf
- Salt to taste
- Pepper powder to taste
- 1 tablespoon tomato paste
- ½ tablespoon unseasoned rice vinegar
- 1 small sprig thyme

Directions

1. Separate the leaves of the cabbage. Place a layer of cabbage leaves at the bottom of a small casserole dish that can be used over the stovetop. You can also use a small pot.
2. Place a pot with water over medium heat. When water begins to boil, dip the remaining cabbage leaves in the boiling water for 1-2 minutes. Drain and dry the leaves with paper towels.
3. Add pork, pork rinds, celery, salt, pepper, nutmeg, onion and egg into a bowl and mix well using your hands.
4. Place a layer of blanched cabbage leaves in the casserole dish.

5. Spread a layer of the meat mixture.
6. Repeat the layering of cabbage and meat mixture until it is over but make sure the topmost layer is of cabbage.
7. Whisk together in a bowl, soy sauce, tomato paste, bay leaf, vinegar and thyme and pour over the casserole.
8. Pour broth on top. The broth should just cover the cabbage. So if you think the broth is extra, use it in some other recipe.
9. Place the casserole dish over low heat. Place a lid directly touching the cabbage, to prevent the casserole from rising. The lid should be smaller than the casserole dish.
10. Simmer for 40-50 minutes.

Nutritional Information per Serving: Calories: 201g, Carbohydrates: 7g, Protein: 16g, Fat: 11 g

Servings: 4 per person

Ingredients

- 3 eggs
- 1 tablespoon almond flour
- 2 ounces cream cheese
- 1 teaspoon garlic powder
- ¼ teaspoon powdered stevia
- 5 tablespoons coconut oil
- ¼ teaspoon black pepper
- 1 teaspoon salt

Directions

1. Crack the eggs into a mixing bowl and add the cream cheese to it.
2. Whisk the eggs and cheese together thoroughly.
3. Add the salt, pepper and garlic powder to the egg-cheese mixture.
4. Add the stevia and almond flour to the mixture. Beat the contents on high speed for three minutes and set the batter aside.
5. Heat a large pan over medium heat and add a bit coconut oil.
6. Pour two tablespoons of the mixed better into the hot skillet.
7. Allow it to cook for 2 minutes until completely set.
8. Using a spatula, flip the pancake to the other side and cook for one minute.
9. Repeat steps 6 to 8 with the remaining batter.
10. Transfer to a plate and serve hot.

Spinach Almond Stir Fry

Servings: 12 per person

Ingredients

- 1-pound spinach leaves
- 3 tablespoon almond slices
- Salt to taste
- 1 Tablespoon coconut oil for cooking

Directions

1. Place the 1 tablespoon coconut oil into a large container on medium heat.
2. Add in the spinach and let it cook.
3. Once the spinach is cooked, add the salt to taste and stir.
4. Before serving, stir in the almond slices.

Nutritional Information per Serving: Calories: 152g, Carbohydrates: 12g, Protein: 10g, Fat: 8g

Bacon and Chicken Chowder

Servings: 8 per person

Ingredients

- 1 trimmed and sliced leek
- 6 oz. sliced cremini mushrooms
- 1 finely chopped shallot
- 1 med. Thinly sliced sweet onion
- 4 minced garlic cloves
- 4 tablespoons butter
- 2 diced celery ribs
- 1-pound chicken breasts
- 2 cup chicken stock
- 1 cup heavy cream
- 8 oz. cream cheese
- 1-pound bacon
- 1 tablespoon dried thyme
- 1 tablespoon Black pepper
- 1 tablespoon Garlic powder
- 1 tablespoon sea salt

Directions

1. Using the low setting for 1 hr. add the shallot, garlic, leek, mushrooms, celery, onions, one cup of the chicken stock, black pepper, sea salt, and 2 tablespoons of butter. Secure the lid.
2. In a skillet, sear the chicken breasts over the med. High setting on the stovetop using the rest of the butter. It should take approximately 5 minutes Per side. Make sure that they are brown on both sides. Set aside on a platter.
3. Deglaze the pan with the rest of the stock using a rubber spatula. Fold in the chicken. Pour in the cream, garlic powder, thyme, and cream cheese, powder,

thyme, and cream cheese. Combine the mixture until the chunks of cheese are mixed well in the mixture.

4. After the chicken has cooled down, cut it into cubes. Stir it back in with the bacon. Stir, cover, and simmer for 6 to 8 har

5. Serve and enjoy when ready.

Nutritional Information per Serving: Calories: 350 g, Carbohydrates: 7 g, Protein: 23 g, Fat: 26 g

Low-carb garlic chicken

Servings: 4 per person

Ingredients

- 2 pounds chicken drumsticks
- 10 minced garlic cloves
- ½ cup finely chopped fresh parsley
- 2 tablespoons olive oil
- 4 tablespoons butter
- Juice of 1 lemon

Directions

1. Preheat the oven to 450-degrees F
2. Grease the baking tray with 1-tablespoon butter.
3. Place the chicken in the greased baking tray and sprinkle generously with pepper and salt.
4. Now, sprinkle the parsley and garlic over the chicken. Drizzle with the olive oil and lemon juice on the top finally.
5. Bake for 40 minutes until the chicken is roasted and minced garlic turns brown.
6. Reduce the temperature towards the last 10 minutes and let it cook.
7. Transfer the garlic chicken to the plate. Serve warm.

Buttered Brussels Sprouts

Servings: 4 per person

Ingredients

- 2 tablespoons fresh lemon juice
- ½ teaspoon salt
- ¼ cup ghee
- 1-pound brussels sprouts
- Pinch Freshly ground black pepper
- 2 crushed garlic cloves
- 1 med. Sliced white onion
- ¼ cup toasted pine flaked almonds
- ½ cup grated parmesan cheese

Directions

1. Set the oven in advance to 400-degree F.
2. Rinse and quarter the sprouts and add the melted ghee along with a drizzle of lemon juice. Add any other ingredients you like.
3. Bake for 24-35 minute until the outsides are crunchy. Stir occasionally.

Nutritional Information per Serving: Calories: 170 g, Carbohydrates: 10 g, Protein: 8 g, Fat: 12 g

Instant Pot Steamed Crab Legs

Servings: 4 per person

Ingredients

- 4 tablespoons butter, melted
- ¾ cup water
- Lemon juice
- 2-pound frozen carb legs

Directions

1. Start by placing the steamer basket into the instant pot then put the crab legs on it.
2. Add in water and lock the lid in place.
3. Then press manual and set the timer to 2 minutes. Let it cook until the timer goes off then quick release pressure. The crab meat, once cooked, should be bright pink in color.
4. Combine juice with some melted butter then serve.

Nutritional Information per Serving: Calories: 185 g, Carbohydrates: 8 g, Protein: 15 g, Fat: 8 g

Garlic Bacon Wrapped Chicken Bites

Servings: 2 per person

Ingredients

- 1 chicken breast, cut into small bites
- 7-8 thin slices of bacon, cut into thirds
- 3 Tablespoons garlic powder

Directions

1. Preheat oven to 400F and line a baking tray with aluminum foil.
2. Place the garlic powder into a bowl and dip each chicken bit into the garlic powder.
3. Warp each short bacon piece around each garlic chicken bite. Place the bacon enfolded chicken bites on the baking tray. Try to interplanetary them out so they're not touching.
4. Bake for 30-35 minutes until the bacon turns crispy. Turn the pieces after 20 minutes if you can remember.

Nutritional Information per Serving: Calories: 225 g, Carbohydrates: 8 g, Protein: 25 g, Fat: 10 g

Homemade Greek Yogurt

Servings: 4 per person

Ingredients

- ½ cup plain full-fat yogurt
- ½ gallon whole milk

Directions

1. To make Greek yoghurt, line a fine mesh using 3 layers of cheesecloth, then put it in a large bowl.
2. Move the yoghurt to a sieve and allow the liquid whey to drain so that you can get preferred yoghurt consistency. This should take around 4 hours.
3. Chill the yoghurt and then serve.

Nutritional Information per Serving: Calories: 225g, Carbohydrates: 8g, Protein: 22g, Fat: 10g

Crockpot Brownie Bites

Servings: 2 per person

Ingredients

- 2 tablespoons brewed coffee or water
- 1 teaspoon pure vanilla extract
- ½ cup coconut oil melted
- tablespoons coconut milk, unsweetened
- 1 egg
- ½ teaspoon salt
- 1 teaspoon baking soda
- 1 teaspoon baking powder
- 4 tablespoons cocoa powder, unsweetened
- tablespoons coconut sugar
- 12 tablespoons almond flour, blanched

Directions

1. First use coconut oil to grease the slow cooker.
2. Then mix all ingredients and spread them evenly on the cooker.
3. Cook the mixture for 4-5 hours until well cooked through.
4. At this point, allow to cool for 30 minutes then scoop out using a large spoon or cookie scoop. Make it into balls.
5. Scoop the snack with caramel glaze if you like.

Nutritional Information per Serving: Calories: 320 g, Carbohydrates: 20 g, Protein: 9 g, Fat: 20 g

Almond Butter Fudge

Servings: 12 per person

Ingredients

- 1 cup almond butter
- 1 cup coconut oil
- ¼ cup coconut milk
- 1 teaspoon vanilla extract
- Stevia for taste

Directions

1. Melt the almond butter and coconut oil so that they are soft.
2. Blend all the ingredients together well.
3. Pour the mixture into a baking pot and refrigerate for 1-2 hours for it to set.
4. Cut into chunks and serve.

Nutritional Information per Serving: Carbohydrates: 3 g

Guacamole Topped Scrambled Eggs

Servings: 1 per person

Ingredients

- 3 eggs
- 1 tablespoon coconut oil
- ¼ cup guacamole
- Salt to taste

Directions

1. Place the coconut oil into a pot add the eggs and scramble over a low-medium heat.
2. Place the twisted eggs into a container and top with the guacamole. If you want, you can add salt.

Nutritional Information per Serving: Calories: 365 g, Carbohydrates: 7 g, Protein: 20 g, Fat: 5 g

Italian Tomato Salad

Servings: 1 per person

Ingredients

- Minced garlic clove – 1
- Freshly chopped basil – 0.25 cup
- Olive oil – 2 tablespoons
- Balsamic vinegar – 1 tablespoon
- Pepper and salt for taste
- Sliced tomatoes – 2 Pcs
- Fresh arugula – 3 cups
- Cubed mozzarella cheese – 3 oz.

Directions

1. Combine the oil, basil, garlic pepper, salt, and vinegar in a blender. Mix until smooth.
2. Toss the rest of the Ingredients in a salad container.
3. Combine the salad and add the dressing mixture or add it to individual containers for an on-to-go method.
4. You can store this way for up to one day.

Nutritional Information per Serving: Calories: 275, Carbohydrates: 10g, Protein:15g, Fat:20g

Eggs and Steak

Servings: 1 per person

Ingredients

- 3 eggs
- 4 ounces sirloin
- 2 tablespoons butter
- ¼ avocado (sliced into cubes)
- Salt and pepper, to teste

Directions

1. Melt one tablespoon butter in a saucepan over low heat and crack in the eggs into it.
2. Fry the eggs until the yolk get cooked thoroughly and the whites are set
3. Add the required salt and prepper. Mix the contents thoroughly.
4. Heat another pan and cook the sirloin in the remaining butter until the meat is soft and tender.
5. Using the spatula, break the meat into small pieces. Season with salt and pepper, and mix the contents thoroughly.
6. Remove both the pans from heat and mix the contents together in a large bowl.
7. Transfer to a plate and serve with sliced avocado.

Conclusion

We are come to the end of the book. Thank you for reading my book and congratulations for reading until the end of the book.

As far as options go, you won't be short of them when you follow a ketogenic diet because there are just so many recipes that you can prepare. And given that you can leverage on the power of the instant pot in retaining the nutritional information in foods and the fact that the instant pot fastens cooking, you can be sure that you won't have any reason not to eat ketogenic diet friendly recipes. I hope this book has opened your eyes to the endless possible ways through which you can prepare keto friendly meals using an instant pot. Now is your time to take action i.e. choosing any of the recipes here to follow the ketogenic diet like a pro!

Thank you and good luck!

www.ingramcontent.com/pod-product-compliance
Lightning Source LLC
Chambersburg PA
CBHW062050280526
45788CB00003B/1181